HORMONE BALANCED DIET

Natural Ways to Restore Hormone Balance

DR. PRECIOUS ETON

TABLE OF CONTENT

INTRODUCTION

Hormonal irregular characteristics can bring on some issues from fruitlessness to diabetes, however certain food varieties can assist with keeping your hormones adjusted and your body working appropriately. We'll show you the foods to focus on for optimal hormonal health. Whenever we contemplate what to eat to feed our bodies, hormones may not be top 100% of the time. However, our hormones take a vital part in our bodies. Hormones are substance couriers that are important for the endocrine framework and help with development and advancement, digestion and assimilation, fruitfulness, stress and mind-set and that's only the tip of the iceberg. Whenever hormones escape balance, to an extreme or too little are produced or something slows down flagging pathways, it can prompt issues like diabetes, weight reduction or gain, or barrenness, among different issues. A sound eating routine can assist with keeping hormones in a state of harmony. Here is an outline of what your hormones control and which food sources keep them adjusted.

CHAPTER ONE

What Diet Means For Hormones

Hormone synthesis and secretion can be influenced by direct acts on the gut, neurological responses, changes in the concentration of different metabolites in the blood, or changes in circulating gut hormone levels. What we consume has an impact on hormone synthesis and signaling pathways. Our hormones are comparable to solid fats such as olive oil nuts, seeds and avocado, as well as abundant fiber from soil-based products and high-quality proteins such as fish, meat and egg. Conversely, pesticides, liquor and fake sugars can adversely affect hormones.

You want an adequate number of calories as well. Women's bodies, in particular, are extremely sensitive to scarcity. If your system doesn't feel like it's receiving sufficiently, it will slow down the production of sex hormones. Your body doesn't have the foggiest idea about the distinction between a conflict or starvation or another weight reduction diet you're following.

CHAPTER TWO

The Most Effective Method to Know Whether Hormones Are Imbalanced

Hormones play a very important role in the overall well-being of the human body. As a response, a variety of indications and symptoms may point to a hormonal imbalance. Whatever hormones or glands are failing will define the signs and symptoms you experience. Any of the preceding signs or symptoms can be caused by common hormonal disorders that influence both men and women:

- Inexplicable, and at times unexpected, slimming down
- Fatigue
- Muscle wasting
- Pains, tenderness, and stiffness in the muscles

- You may experience pain, rigidity, or inflammation in your joints.
- heart rate increase or decrease
- Constipation or more frequent bowel movements higher sensitivity to cold or heat sweating
- Urination on a regular basis enhanced thirst and hunger while lowering sex desire depression.
- Anxiety manifests itself as nervousness, anxiety, or restlessness.
- Eyesight problems
- Infertility
- Dry skin puffy face rounder face purple or pink stretch marks thinning hair or fine, brittle hair

Remember that these are general symptoms that don't always indicate a hormonal imbalance.

Female signs and symptoms

The most common hormonal disorder in women of reproductive age is polycystic ovarian syndrome (PCOS). During these times, your usual hormonal cycle also changes:

- Puberty \pregnancy
- Breastfeeding \menopause

Symptoms specific to only females with hormonal imbalance include:

- Missed periods, periods that have halted, or periods that occur regularly are all examples of heavy or irregular periods.
- Acne seen on the face, chest, or upper back hirsutism, or excessive hair on the face, chin, or other parts of the body hair lossDarkening of the skin, particularly in the wrinkles of the neck, the groin, and beneath the breasts
- Tags on the skin

- Dryness of the vaginal canal
- Night sweats
- headaches
- vaginal atrophy
- pain during sex

Male signs and symptoms

Testosterone is a crucial component in male growth. It can create a number of symptoms if you aren't developing enough testosterone. Chemical imbalance in male adults expresses itself in the following ways:

- Erectile dysfunction gynecomastia, or the development of breast tissue breast tenderness (ED)
- Hair growth on the beard and on the body is slowing down.
- Muscle loss, often known as osteoporosis, problems concentrating hot flushes

However, the most ideal way to know without a doubt is to get tested.

CHAPTER THREE

How Hormones Work in Your Body

In the human body, there are over 200 hormones. Estrogen, testosterone, cortisol, insulin, leptin, ghrelin and thyroid hormones are the most normally known. These are intertwined with metabolism, fertility, and mental health.

Digestion

1. Insulin: Insulin is set free from the pancreas after you eat and takes sugar (glucose) from the blood to cells for energy. Insulin is likewise the hormones answerable for putting away additional sugar as fat.
2. Leptin: This is liberated from fat cells and aids with hunger control, maintain your weight and tell your mind that you are satisfied. It's commonly referred to as "satiety hormones."

3. Ghrelin: This substance, often known as "hunger hormones," is responsible for energizing your desire.
4. Thyroid hormones: Triiodothyronine (T3) and thyroxine (T4) assist with managing weight, energy, temperature, development of hair, skin, nail etc.

Reproductive System

1. Estrogen: This is the female sex chemical that prompts changes during pubescence and controls feminine cycle, keep up with pregnancy, hold cholesterol under tight restraints and keep bones solid.
2. Testosterone: The male sex hormone that causes desire for sex, bone thickness, and muscular strength to increase throughout pubescence (in all kinds of people).

Stress and Mood

1. Cortisol: Cortisol is transported in the middle of stress and expands pulse. An excessive amount of isn't great for your wellbeing, and it's frequently alluded to as the "stress chemical."
2. Adrenaline: Our "acute stress" chemical is delivered in the midst of stress and expands pulse.
3. Melatonin: This substance is released in the evening and prepares the body for sleep. It's regularly called our "rest initiating chemical."

CHAPTER FOUR

Best Food Sources for Hormonal Balance

Cruciferous vegetables

Cruciferous veggies, particularly broccoli sprouts and broccoli, are geniuses at assisting our livers with making do with estrogen in a competent and solid manner. Sprouts, cauliflower, kale, Brussels and cabbage are cruciferous vegetables also. Consuming them consistently is one method for shielding you from creating estrogen-prevailing tumors, Broil them with a sprinkle of olive oil, which helps increment ingestion of nutrients A, D, E and K or attempt them in our broccoli-cauliflower soup.

Salmon and tuna fish

Fat and cholesterol are the structure squares of hormones. You really want sufficient cholesterol to make sex hormones like estrogen and testosterone. The idea is to choose omega-3-rich fats and limit saturated fats (and clear out trans fats). Salmon, canned tuna fish, pecans, flaxseed, olive oil, avocados and chia seeds are high in omega-3 unsaturated fats.

Salmon likewise balances out your yearning hormones and is high in vitamin D, which manages female testosterone levels. The great fats in fish work on generally speaking hormonal correspondence. The endocrine framework utilizes hormones to speak with the mind, which thus supports our mind-set and gives us better mental abilities."

Avocados

Avocados are stacked with beta-sitosterol, which can decidedly influence blood cholesterol levels and assist with adjusting cortisol, the plant sterols in avocados likewise impact estrogen and progesterone, the two hormones answerable for managing ovulation and feminine cycles. The blend of fat and fiber in avocados expanded hormones that advance satiety, including peptide YY (PYY), cholecystokinin (CCK) and glucagon-like peptide 1 (GLP-1). Add a large portion of an avocado to breakfast or lunch to assist you with remaining full for a really long time, or utilize avocado in these sound avocado plans.

Leafy foods (ideally natural)

There are concentrates on that show that even one serving of a high-pesticide organic product or vegetablc (like strawberries) adversely affects richness. Numerous pesticides go about as chemical disruptors, meaning they either copy hormones in your body or they influence the activities of your own hormones. It is critical to avoid synthetics that disrupt the endocrine system, and it is well accepted that glyphosate, for example, is an endocrine disruptor. You can significantly reduce your exposure to glyphosate by maintaining a natural diet. Likewise, the advantages of eating foods grown from the ground far offset not eating them on the off chance that you can't stand to eat natural. Limit openness assuming you can, yet realize that all leafy foods are plentiful in nutrients, minerals and cancer prevention agents.

High-fiber starches

Natural products, vegetables and entire grains. Eating an eating regimen high in fiber can assist with cleaning abundance hormones off of the body. Fiber, as well as lignans, which are plentiful in flaxseed, works with restricting and evacuation of unbound dynamic estrogens. Focus on making a major chunk of your plate non-dull veggies for suppers and a fourth of your plate bland vegetables like potatoes or whole grains. Root vegetables like carrots, yams and squashes can be useful, alongside entire grains and beans, including some starch at supper might assist with controlling the hormones melatonin and cortisol as well. Truth be told, some carbs can truly assist with alleviating raised cortisol levels.

Prebiotics and probiotics

Probiotics are the great microbes that live in the gut, while prebiotics are sinewy food sources those microorganisms grub on to prosper. The gut is the biggest endocrine organ in the body and blends and secretes in excess of 20 hormones that assume a part in craving, satiety and digestion. Instances of prebiotic food sources incorporates: crude garlic, onions, leeks, oats and so forth Instances of probiotics incorporate kimchi, grasshopper beans, green pea, yogurt and so forth

CHAPTER FIVE

Most Awful Food Sources for Chemical Equilibrium

To minimize hormone imbalances, eat fewer processed foods, fried meals, sugar and artificial sweeteners, and drink less alcohol. Artificial sweeteners, according to research, may modify our gut bacteria, affecting the balance of hunger and satiety, as well as the hormones leptin and ghrelin.

Alcohol disrupts a number of hormonal systems, including blood sugar regulation and estrogen metabolism. The consumption of alcoholic beverages has been related to an increased risk of breast cancer and other malignancies. If you're a woman, restrict yourself from drinking more than one drink per day, and if you're a guy, restrict from drinking more than two drinks per day.

CHAPTER SIX

Exercise, Stress and Rest

Notwithstanding keeping feelings of anxiety low, getting satisfactory rest, having a solid eating regimen, and exercising consistently are on the whole necessities for hormonal balance. Lack of sleep is connected to low testosterone in men, and absence of rest obstructs leptin and ghrelin, henceforth, why you will generally want carbs and every one of the tidbits when you're worn out.

Constant pressure prompts raised degrees of cortisol, which smothers the stomach related and safe frameworks and can cause hypertension. Cortisol additionally prompts carbohydrate cravings. Work out, meditation, rest and eating chocolate help levels of norepinephrine and serotonin. Norepinephrine helps energy, and serotonin is the "feel good" hormone

CHAPTER SEVEN

Conclusion

Hormones have an impact on many aspects of life, including growth and development, metabolism, digestion, fertility, stress, mood, energy, appetite, and weight. Hormone balance is maintained by consuming diets enrich in grain products, healthy fats, fruits, protein and vegetables. Obesity, diabetes, infertility, and cancer can all be caused by not getting enough overall calories, good fats, or fiber in your diet. Sleep deprivation, stress, alcohol, and processed meals can all affect hormones in some way, either directly or indirectly, by affecting the gut microbiome, which keeps hormones in check.

www.ingramcontent.com/pod-product-compliance
Ingram Content Group UK Ltd.
Pitfield, Milton Keynes, MK11 3LW, UK
UKHW022008190726
13853UKWH00004B/1803

9 798419 510425